Brain Fuel

Supercharge Your Brain, Improve Memory and Lose Weight Eating Genius Foods

Copyright 2018 by Brain Fuel Systems - All rights reserved.

This document is geared towards providing exact and reliable information in regards to the topic and issue covered. The publication is sold with the idea that the publisher is not required to render an accounting, officially permitted, or otherwise, qualified services. If advice is necessary, legal or professional, a practiced individual in the profession should be ordered.

- From a Declaration of Principles which was accepted and approved equally by a Committee of the American Bar Association and a Committee of Publishers and Associations.

In no way is it legal to reproduce, duplicate, or transmit any part of this document in either electronic means or in printed format. Recording of this publication is strictly prohibited and any storage of this document is not allowed unless with written permission from the publisher. All rights reserved.

The information provided herein is stated to be truthful and consistent, in that any liability, in terms of inattention or otherwise, by any usage or abuse of any policies, processes, or directions contained within is the solitary and utter responsibility of the recipient reader. Under no circumstances will any legal responsibility or blame be held against the publisher for any reparation, damages, or monetary loss due to the information herein, either directly or indirectly.

Respective authors own all copyrights not held by the publisher.

The information herein is offered for informational purposes solely and is universal as so. The presentation of the information is without a contract or any type of guarantee assurance.

The trademarks that are used are without any consent, and the publication of the trademark is without permission or backing by the trademark owner. All trademarks and brands within this book are for clarifying purposes only and are the owned by the owners themselves, not affiliated with this document.

Table of Contents

Introduction

Chapter 1: What Weakens Our Brain?

    Food as Fuel: The Risks of Choosing Low-Quality Fuel

    The Effects of Stress on the Brain

    Nutrition and the Brain

    The Direct Connection Between the Digestive Tract, Your Body, and Your Brain

Chapter 2: The 7 Worst Foods for Your Brain

    Trans Fats

    Mercury-Rich Fish

    Sugary Drinks

    Refined Carbohydrates

    Aspartame

    Heavily Processed Foods

    Alcohol

Chapter 3: Supercharge Your Mitochondria

    Eating Tips to Boost Mitochondrial Health

    Best Foods to Supercharge the Mitochondria

Chapter 4: Boost Brain Health

    The Ketogenic Diet

    The Importance of Ketones

Other Foods That Boost Brain Health

Chapter 5: Memory Rescue

   How Good Fats Benefit the Brain

   The Incredible Power of Antioxidants

   Fish Oil and Brain Health

Chapter 6: Eat Fat, Lose Weight

   The Science Behind a Low-Carb, High-Fat Diet

   Choosing Good Fats

Chapter 7: Brain Boosting Super-Herbs and Nootropics

   Natural Nootropics: What Are They

   10 Brain-Boosting Super-Herbs and Nootropics

Conclusion

Introduction

When was the last time you had fast food or a heavily processed meal? Think back to the way that you felt afterward. Did you feel energized and ready to tackle the rest of the tasks ahead of you or did you feel bloated, tired and fatigued? While most people realize the toll that regularly eating unhealthy foods can take on their waistline, many do not realize that the foods also take a toll on their ability to think clearly. Poor dietary choices can affect your ability to retain information and think quickly and rationally.

By contrast, the right foods will act as fuel for your brain. They will give you the ability to think clearly and maximize your memory. As an added benefit, many also have properties that can help you lose or maintain weight.

In this book, we will go over the psychology of food and how it interacts with your brain to provide the fuel you need for function. After discussing the major differences in how different types of foods affect the brain, we'll break down the benefits of different food groups by chapter and how each food group maximizes your brain health, helping you retain and recall information and supercharge your brain. You'll learn about how to use fats to fuel the brain and help weight loss efforts, how mitochondrial health impacts brain health, the best and worst foods for your brain, nootropics that improve brain health, and more. With this information, you'll find yourself prepared to tackle any task or challenge that you may have in the day ahead.

You'll learn that a lot of the problems with the foods that we eat is the low amount of nutritional value compared to the calories. Not only will the foods mentioned throughout this book provide a healthy stream of antioxidants, healthy fats, vitamins, and minerals to power your brain, these nutrient-dense foods contain calories that count. This can help you maintain or lose weight without even trying.

Are you ready to start making your diet work for you? Keep reading!

Chapter 1: What Weakens Our Brain?

Many people in today's society lead busy lifestyles. Things like employment, meeting the demands of family life, getting an education, and finding time to relax all take a toll on the ability to eat well. Unfortunately, not being able to eat well can mean eating ready-made or fast food. Often, these foods are high in calories but low in the nutrients that your body needs to function at its peak capabilities.

Food as Fuel: The Risks of Choosing Low-Quality Fuel

When you eat unhealthy or heavily processed foods, it is the same as putting low-quality fuel in your engine. Even though it may still get you where you need to go eventually, it is going to make this trip with less efficiency and may cause damage to your car. Just think about the problems that sludgy oil can have—it distributes flecks of metal through your engine and exhaust system, causing what can become permanent damage. The same is true of the foods you eat. If you eat a diet high in sugar, for example, it causes promotes the oxidation of cells and creates free radicals. Diets high in sugar also promote inflammation through the body and damage your body's ability to regulate insulin levels. Some studies have even linked high sugar consumption to worsening symptoms of mood disorders like depression. Additionally, the inflammatory cells and free radicals may move around in the brain, circulating and causing injury to the brain tissue.

The Effects of Stress on the Brain

Inside every cell in the body are mitochondria. The energy from the foods you eat fuel the mitochondria, which in turn provides energy and information to the cell. The mitochondria exist even in the most primitive bacteria, being the cell that makes up all living things.

The mitochondria are a necessary part of our genetic makeup. Recent research, however, shows that the mitochondria are heavily influenced by stress. This means that when you are under psychological stress of some kind, it can trigger a multisystemic stress response. This stress oxidizes the cells and can result in free radicals. It also triggers inflammatory and metabolic reactions and has effects on the neuroendocrine system. What this means is that when you are under psychological stress, your entire is body stressed—from your brain cells to your organs.

It is important to mention that on its own, stress does not cause disease. The ability to deal with stressful situations can help people propel themselves to success and protect them from possible dangers. This is a system that has evolved since the beginning of time. When stress becomes overwhelming, however, it wreaks havoc on a cellular level. It promotes disease that will last as long as the stress does—sometimes through your entire lifespan.

When Stress Becomes Harmful
Everyone experiences stress, a condition defined by the National Institute of Mental Health as 'the brain's response to any demand.' The problem lies in the

intensity and duration of the stress, as well as the steps people take to treat it. Some types of stress are short-term. For example, arguing with a friend or loved one might cause temporary stress. Other people experience long-term stress, from circumstances like having a demanding job, dealing with financial struggles, or managing long-term illness. Regarding treatment, consider 'normal' responses to stress. One person who works a high-stress job may unwind after work by going to the gym. This gives them a healthy outlet and can clear the mind. Another person may 'treat' their stress by going for a few beers after work. This does not deal with the stress in any way, it just numbs it. There is also the added stress and poor health effects that result from drinking regularly.

When stress is not dealt with in a healthy way and when it is caused by a long-term event, it causes 'toxic' or 'chronic' stress. It is chronic stress that is most toxic to the health of the body and mind. At the moment that a stressful event occurs, the amygdala is activated and it signals to the hypothalamus that it is in stress. Then, the hypothalamus communicates this message with the rest of the body, giving it the energy that it would need in for a critical 'fight or flight' response. The fight or flight response has existed since the beginning of man. It is an ingrained response to danger—like facing a bear in the wild—where the only options are to fight the bear or try to outrun it. While the average stresses that people experience in their day-to-day lives are vastly different from those experienced by primitive man, the reaction is the same.

The signal sent out by the amygdala in times of stress triggers the fight or flight response. The body responds physiologically. Heart rate increases to push oxygen and hormones through the blood faster, providing the energy needed for fighting or running. The five senses become more alert, trying to take in information that can be used for survival. Someone who thinks someone is in their house is more likely to hear a slight noise because their hearing is sharpened. The body takes in extra oxygen and a surge of adrenaline prepares the body. The hormone cortisol is also released, which restores energy levels as they are depleted.

When people deal with chronic stress, however, the body cannot release all the cortisol that it is producing in these times of 'danger.' The brain starts to lose its ability to function properly in many ways. Synaptic signals are disrupted, meaning the brain cannot communicate properly between neurons. People may begin avoiding social situations because their synaptic disruption also disrupts their sociability. Studies have even proven that stress shrinks the prefrontal cortex, reducing its total size and killing brain cells. As the prefrontal cortex is the center of learning and memory, it can make it difficult to learn new things and remember old ones. Furthermore, stress increases the size of the amygdala, making the brain more receptive to stress and causing more severe problems in the future.

Mitochondrial Dysfunction and Stress

When learning about biology and basic genetic make-up, one of the first things students learn is about the presence of DNA, cells and mitochondria. The mitochondria are commonly referred to as the 'powerhouse' of the cell. It is critical in the production of adenosine triphosphate or ATP. ATP is the primary source of energy in all live organisms, from trees and plants to animals and people. In humans, it is responsible for synthesizing chemicals, communicating nerve impulses and contracting muscles.

When psychological stress is experienced, it triggers reactions all through the body. Inflammation and cellular response cause a general inability to function, resulting in extra fatigue and other symptoms, generally those that are commonly found in chronic diseases. Not only are the mitochondria affected by this stress, but it also causes an outward ripple of symptoms through the body. The cells cannot perform their functions and the body burns itself out as it tries to continue the processes it needs to survive without enough energy.

You can see the connection between mitochondria disorder and functioning by considering looking at chronic disease. People with mitochondrial dysfunction often experience advanced aging and fatigue. Mitochondrial dysfunction also commonly occurs in neurodegenerative diseases including Friedreich's ataxia, Huntington's disease, Parkinson's disease, Alzheimer's disease, and amyotrophic lateral sclerosis. It is also apparent in chronic fatigue syndrome, chronic infections, cancer, musculoskeletal disease, psychiatric conditions, neurobehavioral conditions, cardiovascular diseases, gastrointestinal conditions, diabetes and metabolic syndrome, and autoimmune disorders.

In some people, however, mitochondrial dysfunction does not occur as a symptom. It occurs as a primary condition that disrupts cellular function. It slows down cell processes, causes inflammation, and speeds aging in many areas of the body—including the brain. Mitochondrial dysfunction often works with oxidative stress and can cause many problems in the future, including metabolic disorder, advanced aging, cancer, and age-related neurodegenerative disorder. In the brain, it affects memory and the preservation of brain cells over time. Mitochondrial dysfunction and disease can cause any number of effects in the body since the mitochondria are found in all cells of the body. This is one of the reasons it is so hard to diagnose. By providing your body and mind with proper nourishment, you can form the necessary building blocks for cellular health and to prevent damage caused by mitochondrial dysfunction and oxidative stress.

Sleep, Nutrition, and the Brain

There is a direct connection between the foods that you eat and how well your brain functions. The brain requires a constant supply of energy to control your heartbeat and breathing, process information from your senses, form thoughts, and store memories. It is even at work while you sleep, taking the time to catch up on sorting and storing information rather than resting. This is the reason that proper sleep is so critical to brain health. People who fail to get adequate sleep experience disruptions in how well their brain sends and receives messages. Research shows that poor sleep habits result in difficulty performing cognitive tasks, including remembering and storing information. It also advances neurodegenerative disease. There is a protein developed in the brain called beta-amyloid. It is toxic and has been found to have links to amnesia, Alzheimer's disease, and neurodegeneration. This is produced through the day, but the brain has time to wash it away when your body is resting at night. If the brain does not have time to eliminate this protein, it builds up and increases the chance of developing dementia and Alzheimer's later in life.

The reason that we need sleep is that being awake takes a mental and physical toll on the body and mind. The average person has a shelf-life of about 16 hours, meaning they can be awake for 16 hours before it starts taking a toll on their body. After that, the body begins slowing down and the brain starts to lose its functioning. One study even showed that after 19-20 hours without sleep, the brain is so impaired that someone driving has the same level of impairment as a drunk driver.

In addition to providing your brain the rest it needs to thrive, it is important to provide it with the fuel it needs to function. When you eat a poor diet, your mitochondria become tired faster. They are not getting enough fuel, so they have to work over time. This means your body and brain may tire out after less than 16 hours of functioning.

All the tasks carried out by the brain require a steady supply of fuel. When you make poor choices on where to get this fuel, your brain is left searching for the nutrients that it needs to maintain this constant state of functioning. Think of your brain as an engine in an expensive car. While you could just throw whatever gasoline was available in it, the car is going to run best when it is given premium fuel. This premium fuel keeps your engine running at peak function. Likewise, giving your brain healthy food supercharge the mitochondria. They give your brain the fuel it needs to thrive, carrying out daily tasks with ease. This helps prevent disease in the future and keeps your energy stores filled, preventing effects like premature aging, fatigue, and damage to cells.

Building a Healthy Diet for Your Brain

There are many elements of nutrition that impact the brain. Like a car, the brain needs certain vitamins, minerals, fats, and other nutritional elements to run at peak functioning. It does not just need gas—it also needs brake fluid, oil, and countless other parts to run efficiently. There are different elements of the foods that you eat that come into play, each of them benefiting the body and brain in a specific way.

Building a healthy diet for your brain means including all the elements that include its functioning. As you continue to read this book, you'll find that it will be divided into different chapters based on food groups and which foods in these groups are best for promoting brain health. You'll also learn about foods that are harmful to brain health, such as those that cause inflammatory reactions through the body.

Not only will these foods improve your ability to perform cognitive tasks, but they will also nourish your body. There is even a chapter on how to use fats to lose weight—the same fats that boost the overall health of your brain. This information can be a lot to take in, especially if you have poor dietary habits already. However, when you continue to eat heavily-processed, convenient foods, you are doing your body and brain a disservice. You are decreasing your vitality, increasing the likelihood of disease, and generally decreasing your quality of life.

Chapter 2: The 7 Worst Foods for Your Brain

It can be said, without a doubt, that the brain is the most important organ in the body. Few people realize the impact that their dietary choices have on their brain. Certain foods make the brain run sluggishly, while others impact memory and mood, and increase the risk of dementia. We'll discuss the seven worst foods for your brain in a moment. For now, we'll take a look at the brain-gut connection and why it's so important to make good choices for your digestive system.

The Direct Connection between the Digestive Tract, Your Body, and Your Brain

In recent years, the phrase 'the brain in your gut' has become more popular in terms of food psychiatry and the way that foods affect the brain. As scientists learn more about the microorganisms that live in the digestive tract and their overall effect on brain health, more is understood about what the brain needs to function at peak capacity.

Within the gut, the enteric nervous system (ENS) runs from the rectum to the esophagus. The ENS is made up of two thin layers, each consisting of over 100 million nerve cells. These nerve cells won't necessarily help you do your taxes or figure out how to overcome a problem at work, but they are critical for brain functioning. The ENS communicates closely with the brain, being guided in the way that it digests food. The brain relays and absorbs information from the ENS, then decides which enzymes to release to break down food. It is also responsible for the release of nutrients into the bloodstream, making it a critical element of both nutrient absorption and waste elimination.

The ENS, therefore, plays a major role in the availability of nutrients to the brain. To keep the ENS in the digestive tract (and the brain) functioning efficiently, it is necessary to provide it with the foods that it needs. The foods that your body needs are not those that are calorie-dense, low-nutrient choices that have become common in western diets. Instead, it involves eating foods that contain probiotics, antioxidants, and the vitamins and minerals necessary to provide your brain with energy.

While the effects of each of the foods in this chapter differ, they do have something in common. Each of them inhibits gut health in some way. When they pass through the digestive tract, it does harm to the body. It is important to think of the body as a whole ecosystem. When you make poor food choices, it feeds the 'bad' side of this ecosystem and helps create an environment where bacteria, illness and inflammation can thrive. By contrast, eating nutrient-dense foods and making choices that nourish the body in a good way improves gut health, thus improving the health of your brain, immune system, digestive tract, heart, and other areas.

Foods That Harm Brain Health

Trans Fats

What many people hear is that a diet high in fats is good for their brain. However, not all fats have the same chemical makeup or the same effects on your body. One of the most detrimental types of fat for brain health is trans fats. While some trans fats occur naturally in dairy and meat products, it is the ones that are made from hydrogenated vegetable oils that harm your health. They are commonly found in snack foods, prepared cakes, margarine, shortening, frosting, and prepackaged cookies.

While the research on trans fats is mixed, there are several studies that have shown people who consume high levels of trans fats have lower brain volume and poorer memory. Eventually, they may also be at risk for cognitive decline and Alzheimer's disease. Unsaturated fats, on the other hand, have been shown to increase cognitive decline.

Mercury-Rich Fish

While fatty fish are often recommended for improving brain health and cognitive function, there are dangers associated with consuming fish that contain too much mercury. Mercury is a heavy metal that works as a neurological poison in the body. It is accumulated and stored in animal tissue, making predatory fish with long lifespans a major source of mercury.

Even though eating 2-3 servings of fish each week can improve brain health, eating mercury-rich fish has the opposite effect. Mercury is not easily removed as waste by the body. Instead, it accumulates in different areas of the body, concentrating in the liver, kidneys, and brain. In pregnant women, mercury commonly accumulates in the fetus and placenta as well, which can be harmful to the fetus by damaging brain development, destroying the cell components and even causing developmental deficits and delays like cerebral palsy.

Some of the fish typically high in mercury are shark, king mackerel, tuna, swordfish, tilefish, and orange roughie. While children and pregnant woman should not consume high-mercury fish, others may eat one serving per week—but only a single serving. If you are catching and eating freshwater fish, it may be a good idea to get samples tested from the water or fish you catch there—this will stop you from eating mercury and other contaminants that may result from local factory runoff.

Sugary Drinks
Some of the popular beverage choices that are high in sugar include fruit juice, sports drinks, soda, and energy drinks. These are harmful to the body as a whole, causing your blood sugar to skyrocket, increasing the risk of type 2 diabetes, and boosting the risk of heart disease. The biggest risk comes from the high-fructose corn syrup, which is generally made of 55% fructose and 45% glucose. When high-fructose corn syrup is consumed in large amounts, it can cause high blood fats, arterial dysfunction, high blood pressure, diabetes, and obesity. These increase the risk of metabolic system and create free radicals and inflammation that destroy healthy brain cells and result in dementia. If you want variety outside of water, try unsweetened coffee or tea, unsweetened dairy products, or vegetable juice.

Refined Carbohydrates
While there are grain-rich products available, refined carbohydrates come from grains that have undergone heavy processing, often made using white flour. Refined

carbohydrates break down much more quickly than those that have not been refined, which gives them a high glycemic index. The glycemic index is used to determine how quickly foods are digested and used by the body. When they are digested too fast, like refined carbohydrates are, it results in blood sugar spikes.

Several studies have proven that it only takes a single high-glycemic meal to impair memory abilities in children and adults. One reason these memory difficulties may happen is that refined carbohydrates inflame the hippocampus, an area of the brain responsible for sending at signals regarding hunger and fullness and a critical part of the memory process. Additionally, the inflammation that results from eating refined carbohydrates has been proven to create a higher risk for degenerative brain diseases like dementia and Alzheimer's.

Aspartame
One of the things that people commonly do when they are trying to lose weight is cut sugar out of their diet. However, many sugar-free products include an artificial sweetener called aspartame. There has been a lot of controversial research on aspartame, but several have indicated that aspartame causes behavioral and cognitive problems.

Aspartame contains several components, including aspartic acid, methanol, and phenylalanine. The chemical makeup of phenylalanine allows it to cross the blood-brain barrier and disrupt neurotransmitter production. The other problem comes from the classification of aspartame as a chemical stressor. This increases how vulnerable the brain is to oxidative stress. Some of the studies report that aspartame has to be consumed at high amounts for these effects to be seen, however, it is best to cut these artificial sweeteners from your diet altogether.

Heavily Processed Foods
Many people turn to heavily processed foods when they are looking for a quick, cheap alternative to eating. Unfortunately, these heavily processed foods are often high in salt, sugar, and added fats. These are all known for causing weight gain, which makes visceral fat accumulate around the organs. This visceral fat has been proven in several studies to damage healthy brain tissue. Additionally, the decrease of healthy brain tissue can indicate the beginning of metabolic syndrome.

Another major factor in the decrease of brain health comes from the poor nutritional content of highly processed foods. The lack of nutrition and high amount of calories cause fat gain. Additionally, the dangerous ingredients result in free radicals and oxidation that harm healthy cells in the body. There are several studies that have linked poor eating of processed foods to low memory. One showed that a diet high in processed red meats and fried foods result in lower memory and learning skills. Another showed that baked beans, fried foods, red meat, and processed meats cause inflammation in the brain and a significant decline in reasoning resulted over ten years.

Studies in rats showed that the problem may stem from the way processed food interact with the blood-brain barrier. They reduce the production of a molecule called BDNF, or brain-derived neurotrophic factor. The BDNF is found in the hippocampus, making it an important part of long-term memory, the growth of new neurons, and learning.

Alcohol

Alcohol does not always harm the brain. It can be enjoyable to drink with friends or have a glass of wine with a meal. However, if you are constantly consuming alcohol, it can have detrimental effects on the brain. Some of the known effects of chronic alcohol use on the brain include the disruption of neurotransmitters, metabolic changes, and reduction in brain volume. Another problem is the lack of Vitamin B1. Most alcoholics are deficient in this vitamin, which can cause Wernicke's encephalopathy, which may become Korsakoff's syndrome over time. Korsakoff's syndrome results in severe brain damage, including unsteadiness, memory loss, confusion, and eyesight disturbances.

Additionally, alcohol disturbs the natural sleep-wake cycle and can result in poor sleep quality. As the brain requires rest to function, failing to get a restful night of sleep can cause memory problems and impulse control problems. As we learned in the first chapter, it also causes an increase in fatigue. This makes it harder for the mitochondria to function and causes the brain to produce harmful enzymes.

Moderation, Not Deprivation

Take a moment to think about what you have eaten over the past week. Chances are, you have indulged in at least one of the foods in this list. It's important to remember that you are not punishing your body. While choosing unhealthy foods is sometimes a matter of convenience, there is also an addictive factor to consider. Unhealthy foods are comforting because they increase the amount of dopamine in your brain, which is associated with the pleasure center.

The best way to overcome addictions is by cutting them off cold turkey. However, some people may have trouble doing this. For example, people who drink diet soda that is full of artificial sweeteners like aspartame may experience withdrawal symptoms if they kick their habit cold turkey, especially if they drink more than one soda a day. People who can exercise some control over their addiction might better benefit from cutting back on their habit. Instead of going cold turkey from three sodas a day, they might cut back to two sodas per day. Then, they might only drink one soda each day before cutting it out completely. This gives their body time to adjust to the changes and makes it less likely that they will experience withdrawal symptoms.

For people who cannot control their addictive food tendencies, it is best to cut it out together. Alcohol, for example, is something that may need cut out cold turkey for some people. Processed or sugary foods may also need to be cut out completely. This is especially true for people who may think that they need 'just one more' cookie or French fry to satisfy their fix.

Unhealthy Foods and Addiction
It is easy for the mind to become addicted to the taste of processed foods. Think about the relief you feel when you have been slaving away at work and you can eat a salad or cheeseburger instead of cooking something. Consider the satisfaction that comes with ordering pizza or takeout instead of cooking after you have had a long day. Or how someone might eat a pint of ice cream or binge on tacos after they have gone through a breakup.

When this pleasurable sensation is related to eating, it creates a dependence on it in the mind. When you are dealing with food addiction, it may be best to cut out the harmful foods completely. It is the same as an alcoholic that needs to go cold turkey. Here are some symptoms of food addiction:

- Feelings of guilt or shame after eating something (and then eating it again in the future)
- Attempts to hide unhealthy food consumption from others
- You experience cravings for unhealthy foods, even after finishing a nutritious meal
- It is hard to control consumption of unhealthy food, often causing you to overeat
- You eat food until you feel excessively stuffed, but still may not feel satisfied
- You make excuses about why you should give in to a craving
- You have tried to eat healthier and failed, repeatedly
- You understand how unhealthy foods damage your body but continue to eat them

Research shows that certain foods light up the same pleasure center of the brain that drugs do. The saltiness of cheese or potato chips, for example, triggers the release of dopamine. Cheese goes a step further with addiction, as it contains casein. Casein has a by-product of casomorphins, which have the same opiate molecule structure as heroin and other narcotics. They attach to the same areas of the brain, as well. The way that foods interact with our brain can make it hard to stop a craving or kill the desire to binge eat. However, it is possible.

As with any addiction, you'll need to take several steps to eliminate poor food choices from your life. You can start by making a list of your 'trigger' foods, which are those foods that you cannot seem to say 'no' to. Think about the pros and cons of these foods. While they may be pleasurable to eat, they can also cause weight gain and have poor health consequences. Keep this list handy, being sure to refer to it when you find yourself in a tough spot. Breaking your regular habits can also help. If you find yourself wanting to 'treat' yourself after work when you drive by your favorite fast food place, take a different way home. Only bring enough money to work for lunch or pack lunch and leave your debit card at home, so you can't spend money on the food. Keep healthy snacks handy to help you curb cravings and stay full through the day.

For some people struggling with food addiction, speaking to a food therapist might be a good choice. Sometimes, there are underlying problems that cause problems for a person. For example, research shows that children who were forced to finish their entire plate or eat foods they did not like growing up are more likely to have a difficult relationship with food. If you simply cannot kick the habit on your own, get the help you need to stick to healthier eating habits.

Chapter 3: Supercharge Your Mitochondria

The difference in springing out of bed in the morning and dragging yourself through your daily tasks may lie in the way that you treat your mitochondria. As we discussed earlier, the mitochondria provide the power needed for individual cells. They help provide the energy your body needs. Here are some tips you can use to ensure your mitochondria are working for you.

Eating Tips to Boost Mitochondrial Health

Many of the tips that can be used to boost mitochondrial health relate closely to those foods that are bad for the brain. As you consider your diet, try the following things.

1. Cut refined grains and processed sugar from your diet. Mitochondria typically cannot burn sugar carbs fast enough. Instead, they end up stored as fat and can create free radicals.

2. Choose healthy fats. Healthy fats and carbohydrates are the best sources of the raw material mitochondria need to create the ATP that creates energy in the cell. The right fats are best for this, as burning fats results in less radical byproducts. Ideally, you should choose omega-3s for brain health. You'll learn more about which foods are healthy fat in chapters 5 and 6.

3. Enjoy some bone broth. Bone broth can be comforting and warming any time of day. It nourishes the body with a high amount of vitamins and minerals, is rich in amino

acids that make the cells thrive, and protects the lining of the digestive tract.

4. Remove toxins from your diet. Toxins include prepackaged foods that were discussed earlier. However, toxins can also include toxins and pesticides leached into fresh foods while they are growing. To avoid this, avoid factory-farmed and processed foods, by pasture-raised meat products, and buy produce from local organic farms.

5. Enjoy many colors in your diet. Fruits and vegetables get their unique color from phytonutrients that are unique. Sulfur-rich veggies like cabbage, cauliflower, leafy greens should also be included. They help produce an incredibly powerful antioxidant called glutathione.

6. Improve mitochondrial function by doing intermittent fasting. Though many people eat from morning to night, the research shows that it is better to get most of your calories in an 8-hour window. These extra non-eating hours reduce the number of free radicals produced when your mitochondria break down food.

7. Exercising regularly can strengthen mitochondria. When you exercise, it increases blood flow and oxygen. It can also encourage the production of new mitochondria. Studies have shown that there are several types of physical activity that can increase mitochondrial function—running, strength training, and high-intensity interval training.

8. Consider low-level laser therapy (LLLT). This type of treatment uses LEDs or low-level lasers to penetrate the body and stimulate the cells. It has been used in the brain to stimulate and heal brain cells. It also increases ATP

production and reduces oxidative stress that results in free radicals.

Best Foods to Supercharge the Mitochondria

Resveratrol

Resveratrol activates BDNF, which is an important part of learning, memory, and the formation of new cells. This antioxidant compound is most readily found in red wine and grapes. Additionally, resveratrol triggers biochemical reactions because of the way it activates the S1RT1 gene. This can improve the functioning of both your mitochondria and your brain. One study even showed resveratrol could increase lifespan because of its protective abilities over the mitochondria—it was published by Harvard researchers in 2006.

B Vitamins

Oatmeal is one of the best fuels for the brain, especially when you eat it for breakfast. Porridge is one of the few cereals that aren't highly processed and it is rich in fiber that digests slowly in your gut. Not only will it give you the energy you need to get through until lunchtime, but the high fiber content can also help clean out any waste matter that may have accumulated in the gut.

Oats are also a good choice because they contain many of the B-vitamins, which are known for their energy-boosting abilities. They are especially beneficial during times of stress since they nourish the nervous system and become seriously depleted when you are stressed. Many of the B-vitamins are also water soluble, so they are eliminated from the body when there is excess, rather than being stored for later.

B-vitamins should be supplemented into your diet every day. These vitamins are water-soluble, which means that your body does not store them and excess vitamins are eliminated as waste. Additionally, B-vitamins are necessary for your brain to be at its best. When your levels are low, it results in increased irritability and stress, low mood levels, difficulty concentrating, and memory problems.

Among the B-vitamins are Vitamin B12, Vitamin B6, riboflavin, pantothenic acid, biotin, folate (also called folacin or folic acid), niacin, and thiamin. While all of them provide the nourishment that your nervous system needs, Vitamin 6 is especially beneficial to the brain because of the energy it provides for your brain and the role that it plays in the digestive system. Here are a few other foods that are high in Vitamin B:

- Green Vegetables- Most green veggies contain a wide range of vitamins. For example, broccoli, asparagus, spinach, and kale all contain high amounts of riboflavin, pantothenic acid, and folate.
- Meat and Fish- There are several protein groups that you can get B-vitamins from. Pork, for example, contains high levels of niacin, thiamin, and biotin. Beef contains niacin, while chicken and other poultry contain vitamin B12, pantothenic acid, niacin, and riboflavin. Several types of seafood also contain high amounts of B-vitamins, such as haddock, tuna, salmon, clams, and oysters that contain pantothenic acid, biotin, vitamin B6, vitamin B12, and niacin.
- Nutritional Yeast- Nutritional yeast comes in packages that have yellow-orange flakes. Many people say they have a cheese-like taste, so it is

easy to sprinkle them on top of your foods. Nutritional yeast is especially high in vitamin B12.
- Whole Grains- Whole grain carbohydrates are not processed as much as foods like white crackers, pasta, and bread. Many also digest slowly, making them a good choice when you want long-term energy. As an added benefit, many are enriched or fortified, which means they have additional nutritional benefits.
- Fruits- Of the fruits, citrus fruits like lemons, limes, grapefruits, and oranges contain the most folic acid. There are also trace amounts of other B-vitamins, including riboflavin, pantothenic acid, niacin, and thiamin.
- Legumes- For vegetarians, legumes can serve as a healthy source of B-vitamins. The most abundant vitamins in legumes include pantothenic acid, niacin, vitamin B6, thiamin, and folic acid.
- A Few Other Mentions- Some other foods that are full of B-vitamins include sweet potatoes, sunflower seeds, dairy products, eggs, peanuts, peas, and avocados.

Magnesium

Magnesium plays an important role in the regeneration of mitochondria, making them an important part of cell function and boosting brain power. Some of the best food sources include:

- Spinach- Leafy greens, like spinach, have their benefits, but spinach has one of the highest doses of magnesium. It is also rich in vitamin A, vitamin C, and fiber. You can make a salad, blend it in a smoothie, or wilt it on pizza or in soup. Swiss chard is also another good source of magnesium.

- Almonds- Almonds are an easy snack, whether you add them to cereal or yogurt or eat them by the handful. You can also get some magnesium by using almond flour or almond milk in your diet.
- Seeds- While all seeds are a great source of healthy fats, vitamins, and minerals, pumpkin and sunflower seeds are among the best. They are high in minerals that support good concentration and memory, including potassium, selenium, zinc, and magnesium. These same minerals help balance mood and magnesium specifically can help people who struggle with insomnia.
- Banana- A banana has a fair amount of magnesium. It makes a great smoothie base as well, so you could easily throw it into the blender with some spinach and other fruits for a delicious and easy magnesium boost.
- Avocado- An avocado is an easy power-booster for the brain. It is nourishing and full of healthy fats, as well as 60mg of magnesium.

Zinc

The mineral zinc also works as an antioxidant in the body, fighting against inflammation and oxidative stress. It also ensures the health of cytokines, which are proteins that are important in the communication process between different cells. Some foods high in zinc include:

- Cashews and pumpkin seeds- These two nuts/seeds are especially high in zinc. While they only contain about half of the zinc found in grass-fed beef, they are an easy snack that you can use as brain fuel any time.

- Grass-fed Beef- Grass-fed beef is high in zinc, with about 37% of the recommended daily allowance per serving. It is also high in omega-3 fatty acids, which have incredible benefits for the brain.

Coenzyme Q10 (CoQ10)
CoQ10 is naturally produced by the body, but there is a significant decline in production over time. Many people take it as a supplement, as there are only a few food sources of CoQ10. It works as an antioxidant in the way it combats oxidative damage and stress. It also benefits the mitochondria, helping the cells produce the energy they need to carry out functions.

Something to note is that when you take drugs to lower cholesterol, the body does not absorb COQ10 as readily. The body's production generally slows down around age 50. Some good food sources of CoQ10 include-

- Eggs- Eggs are full of nutrition, including CoQ10. Even though egg yolks once got a bad rap for their high cholesterol content, they are the most nutritious part of the egg. They contain many nutrients, protein, and essential fatty acids.

- Tuna, mackerel, and herring- These fish are great sources of CoQ10, whether you eat them canned, smoked, or fresh. Something to note, however, is that you should choose fresh fish from quality areas to avoid mercury exposure.

- Grass-fed Butter- Butter from grass-fed sources has a little more CoQ10 than a serving of eggs. It even remains throughout the cooking process!

- Extra Virgin Olive Oil- This CoQ10 superfood is easy to add to your diet. Use it to make a vinaigrette or marinade, drizzle it over fish or roasted vegetables, or use it to make a sauce for a whole grain pasta dish.

Sulfur
Sulfur is the fourth most abundant mineral found within the human body. It works as an antioxidant and encourages mitochondrial health. They help a strong barrier grow around the mitochondrial, which gives them more defense against free radicals and toxins. While you should enjoy foods high in sulfur, keep in mind that eating too much raw cruciferous vegetables can be painful on the digestive system.

- Kale- Kale fulfills many of your mitochondria's needs. In addition to being incredibly high in sulfur, it contains a high level of antioxidants and can help you meet nutritional requirements for vitamins A, C, and K. Kale contains 10 times the recommended dosage of vitamin K, nearly 100% of vitamin A intake, and about 71% of the recommended amount of vitamin C, which is more vitamin C than is found in an orange. Kale can be sautéed and enjoyed as a side, blended with fruits to make a delicious smoothie, or even slow-roasted to make kale chips. It is also a wonderful source of iron, calcium, and magnesium. As an added benefit, the iron and calcium found in kale are more readily available to the body than the iron and calcium from dairy products and other foods. This is because of its low oxalate content.

- Garlic- Garlic is a superfood for the mitochondria. It is full of antioxidants and sulfur that protect the mitochondria and also has antimicrobial and antibacterial properties. Garlic also packs a flavorful punch.

- Onions- Onions are another versatile vegetable, being able to enhance savory dishes with a mild flavor when they are cooked. They can also be eaten raw in salsas, on sandwiches, and in salads.
- Cabbage- Cabbage is in a wide range of dishes. It can be used in a crisp, tangy coleslaw, be cooked in soups, or added into vegetable stir fries.

Chapter 4: Boosting Brain Health with the Ketogenic Diet

When brain health is involved, a ketogenic diet is known for its incredible ability to boost brain health. We will move onto healthy oils in the next chapter, but for now, we are going to discuss the ketogenic diet, ketones, and some brain-boosting superfoods that can improve your brain health.

The Ketogenic Diet

In the last few decades, the spotlight has been on many low-carb diets. One of the best for brain health is the ketogenic diet, which involves eating a small number of carbohydrate foods and a lot of fatty acids. Once your body and brain adapt, this diet improves your brain function and mental clarity and can help you burn fat.

The key to this diet is allowing the body to enter a state called 'ketosis.' When your body does not have its normal supply of carbohydrates, it enters a state called ketosis where the metabolism burns fatty acids and ketones rather than glucose. Many studies have also shown that a ketogenic diet is helpful for people who suffer from mitochondria dysfunction who want to get their metabolic state back on track. While the research is still being studied, there is also an indication for using ketosis to treat mental health diseases like autism, epilepsy, Alzheimer's, and Parkinson's.

The Importance of Ketones

The state of ketoacidosis that the brain enters when it burns fats for fuel. This state is characterized by a high level of ketones in your brain. Once your body realizes that it is not getting the glucose that it needs to sustain itself, the liver starts producing ketones. The key is not restricting glucose completely—most beginners start by cutting their carbohydrates to just 30-50 grams per day.

The liver uses readily available fatty acids to create ketones. The ketones are fatty acids that are easily used by the brain as fuel. Additionally, once the ketones have started production, the liver continues to convert the stored fatty acids for backup fuel. This means that your brain constantly has a supply of energy to run, rather than just when your blood glucose levels allow it.

The presence of ketones lets your body burn fuel more efficiently. It helps to overcome the problem of low blood glucose levels—as your brain that burns energy on demand is the first to recognize low blood sugar levels. This can even result in a condition known as hypoglycemia in some people, causing system-wide shock.

People who participate in a ketogenic diet should consume fat from a wide variety of sources, as well as fruits and vegetables. The body must receive less than 50 grams of carbohydrates per day to enter and maintain the ketogenic state. However, people who are on the ketogenic diet must test their ketones. If ketones are too high, it can cause the body to enter a dangerous state called ketoacidosis. Ketoacidosis is most easily recognized by the sweet, fruity smell of the breath once the body enters that state. It also causes extreme fatigue and thirst and can lead to coma or death if the ketone levels are not managed.

Carbohydrates, Insulin, and Your Body
To understand why there is so much emphasis on low-carb diets today, it's important to understand what carbohydrates do to your body. Carbohydrates contain molecules of glucose. Glucose is easy to process as energy, so the body resorts to using glucose for energy whenever it is available. The problem is that burning available glucose stops the body from burning the existing fat molecules. Instead, the fat is stored. This can cause weight gain.

Eating carbohydrates also causes the amount of insulin in your bloodstream to skyrocket. The glucose bonds to the glucose and carries it through the body. Since insulin can pass through the cellular membranes, it is the perfect transport mechanism. However, this surge also has negative effects on the body. It disrupts your hunger and satiety hormones, which can make it difficult to know when you are actually hungry. Your body may also become resistant to insulin over time, which means it will produce more when you eat carbohydrates. When this happens, blood sugar levels can rise above normal. This may result in the development of diabetes over time.

Benefits of a Ketogenic Diet

There is a reason that the Keto diet has gotten so much attention in the past few years—it has incredible benefits for the body and mind. As the diet has been researched, more benefits have been discovered. Its many benefits include:

- Weight loss- As your body begins to burn fat cells for fuel, it eats away at the fat stores of your body. Additionally, your body produces a significantly lower amount of insulin when you are on a Keto diet. This lowered insulin allows your hunger and satiety hormones to regulate. This means you get fuller faster and consume fewer calories throughout the day.

- Increased energy- The sudden burst of energy that you feel after drinking a can of soda or eating carbohydrates comes the sudden boost of available fuel from the glucose in the bloodstream. Unfortunately, this leaves as suddenly as it comes and it can leave your body and brain crashing from depleted energy stores. Since the body can rely on its fat stores when it is ketosis, there is a steady supply of energy.

- Better mental focus- When your body starts to produce ketones, they are used by all areas of the body—including the brain. Ketones are used efficiently by the brain while eating a diet high in fats promotes brain health. Additionally, the Keto diet stops spikes in blood pressure that often result in fatigue and mental fog.

- Improved blood sugar levels- People who eat a lot of carbohydrates often experience spikes in their blood sugar throughout the day. It is natural for blood sugar to increase after eating. In people who have diabetes and those who are pre-diabetic, however, this spike can become very dangerous. When blood sugar gets too high, it causes a condition known as hyperglycemia. This can cause frequent urination, fatigue, blurred vision, headache, increased hunger and/or thirst, and sugar in your urine. In addition to improving blood sugar levels, the Keto diet can improve insulin resistance that is common in diabetics and people who experience blood sugar spikes.

- Treatment of epilepsy- Interestingly, the history of the Keto diet goes back to research conducted by Dr. Russell Wilder in the 1920s when he was working at the Mayo Clinic. At the time, his research on the Keto diet was the first of its kind in treating epilepsy. It was used by practitioners as the standard of care for more than a decade until the development of anti-seizure medications in the 1940s. A new interest emerged in the 1990s when a man named Jim Abraham began treating his son Charlie with the Keto diet because conventional medications had been unsuccessful. After having success with the diet, Charlie's family established the Charlie Foundation in 1994 with the purpose of spreading information about how the Keto diet had stopped their son's seizures. Even today, Charlie lives without seizures by eating a Ketogenic diet. This is only one account of success, as many clinical studies have proven the Keto diet is effective in reducing seizures up to 90% or more in many epileptics, especially in children.

- Improved blood pressure and cholesterol- Quality of fat is important on the Keto diet. When you eat healthy fats, it raises the good (HDL) cholesterol and lowers the bad (LDL) cholesterol. Additionally, it improves the balance of triglycerides, especially those associated with the buildup of plaque in the arteries. Other studies have shown low-carb diets decrease blood pressure better compared to other common diets. This decrease in blood pressure may also be influenced by the weight loss that is common on the Keto diet.

- Better skin health- Traditional diets cause inflammation through the body—including in the skin. One study found that eating a high percentage of carbohydrates increase the presence of acne. In another, skin inflammation and lesions were decreased. This included acne, as well as people who suffered from conditions like eczema and psoriasis.

Foods to Eat on a Keto Diet

One of the biggest mistakes that people make when beginning the Keto diet is thinking they can eat as much fat as they want and start to get skinny. It is important to remember that the ideal Keto diet should include healthy fats. When you do consume the small number of carbs required daily, you should eat carbs from fruits, vegetables, and grains instead of flour products and refined sugar. Here are some major "Dos" of the Keto diet:

- Stay hydrated. Water is important for healthy digestion and eliminating toxins from your body. If water gets boring, add stevia-based flavorings. For a non-sweetener alternative, lime or lemon juice makes a good flavoring. Broth and unsweetened tea are other good beverages.

- Eat vegetables. Including colorful vegetables helps you consume a wide range of antioxidants, vitamins, and minerals. While you can eat them fresh or frozen, try not to overcook them. Overcooking them causes some of the nutrients to be released before you consume them. Try to avoid starchy vegetables, particularly those that grow underground. Leafy green vegetables are some of the best for brain health!

- Add nuts and seeds to your diet. Not only are they high in fats and proteins necessary for Keto, but they are also a great source of fuel for the brain. Some nuts and seeds also contain ALA, which is an essential acid for keeping the tissue of the brain healthy.

- Choose full-fat dairy. Partial-fat dairy is usually more processed than full-fat. One of the best sources of protein is hard cheeses, which are minimally processed and lower in calories than other cheeses.

- Choose organic, grass-fed, pasture-raised meat when you can. This is free of antibiotics and growth hormones found in lower-quality meats. While meat doesn't usually have carbohydrates, you should still be cautious about consuming too much protein when on the Keto diet.

- Choose natural sources of oil and fat. Some of the best sources are nuts and meat like beef and fish. You can also supplement with monounsaturated and saturated fats, which are good for brain health. Some good fats include olive oil, full-fat butter, and coconut oil.

Foods to Avoid on a Keto Diet

One of the biggest challenges that some people experience on a Keto diet is eating refined sugars and carbohydrates. While there are some restrictions, the Ketogenic diet is one that offers a lot of variety. It encourages diversity in the foods you choose, especially to balance the micronutrients you are consuming. Even though you should eat a wide range of foods, there are several that should be avoided. These include:

- Low-fat foods- These usually have higher levels of sugar and carbohydrates than full-fat versions.

- Sugary fruits- Large fruits like bananas, oranges, and apples do have health benefits—but they are also high in carbs. Instead, choose low-sugar berries.

- Starches- Starches like yams and potatoes are full of starches that cause the same blood sugar spikes as refined carbs or sugars. You should also avoid oat found in foods like muesli and oats.

- Grains- Grains include any wheat products that cause blood sugar spikes. There are many common foods that fall into this category and that should be avoided, including beer, pasta, bread products, cakes, pasta, pastries, corn, rice, and cereal. Whole grain foods like quinoa buckwheat, rye, buckwheat, and barley should also be avoided.

- Sugar- Sugar is found in beverages, candy, sauces, and many other foods commonly eaten in the Western diet. Read nutrition labels and make educated choices about what you are putting in your body. Some of the other foods on this list can be consumed in moderation, but refined sugars should be eliminated from your diet completely.

Keto and the Brain

After a few days of eating a high-fat, low-carb diet like the Ketogenic diet, many people report a 'boost' of brain energy. While they may experience fatigue as their body transitions, this energy is a type of mental focus and clarity that begins once that transition is complete. This can help them think clearer and better focus on tasks in life.

Not only does Keto boost the energy by providing ketones to the brain, but it also has all the components necessary for brain health. By eating a wide range of antioxidant-rich vegetables, including seasonings and herbs in your diet, and consuming a high level of healthy fats, you can fuel your brain in a way that lets it work at its peak function.

Chapter 5: Memory Rescue

The pressure to be thin is something that has drastically affected certain areas of the world, especially where the media puts pressure on people to look good all the time. This aversion to fats can help some people lose weight, but it also is detrimental to brain health. Not all fats are created equal, and by choosing the right kinds of fats, you can help improve your cognitive function.

How Good Fats Benefit the Brain

The best type of fat for brain health are omega-3 fatty acids. The outer membrane of brain cells is rich in fat, which allows nerve signals to move through the membrane and into the command center of the cell. This is how the brain shares information, both receiving signals from the body and sending out commands. Omega-3s are also used to help create new connections between different nerve cells in the brain, as they cover and protect the new membranes.

Even though the typical American diet is either low in fats or contains too much overall fat, many people are not getting the number of healthy fats they need to maintain strong connections in the brain. One of the problems with this may be that polyunsaturated fats recommended for heart health are not healthy for the brain. Additionally, oils commonly used in cooking like sunflower, corn, and safflower oil do not contain any omega-3s. Instead, they are loaded with omega-6 fats—these can benefit the heart, but they harm brain function.

One of the reasons that people struggle to get enough Omega-3s is because they are quickly used by the body to promote healthy brain function. When you are deficient in omega-3's, it can cause fatigue and memory problems. Another problem is that the body does not produce omega-3 fatty acids on its own. There are natural food sources where they can be eaten. However, some people choose to take fish oil supplements to ensure they are getting the oils they need to promote brain health.

Omega-3 Fatty Acids and Brain Health
The three most important fatty acids for brain health include alpha-linolenic acid (ALA), eicosapentaenoic acid (EPA), and docosahexaenoic acid (DHA). These fats are critical for the healing and health of the brain. At a young age, they play a role in brain development. This is the reason that pregnancy supplements may contain DHA and other components for brain health. One study that followed infants whose mother's took supplements with DHA against a control group showed that those whose mothers had taken the supplement had higher mental processing scores. They also excelled in psychomotor development and hand-eye coordination.

In adults, EPA and DHA are converted to work with different areas of the body. DHA is a critical building block of tissue found in the retina of the eye and brain. It also plays a critical role in the production of neural transmitters, including phosphatidylserine, which is critical for proper brain function. One study carried out by the University of California assessed the potential role of EPA and DHA in clinical applications using double-blind, controlled, and randomized trials. Results showed that there are benefits for DHA and EPA supplementation for bipolar disorder, major depressive disorder, schizophrenia, borderline personality disorder, Huntington's disease, Alzheimer's, attention-deficit hyperactive disorder, dyslexia, autism, aggression, and dyspraxia.

ALA is another fatty acid that plays critical roles in brain health. Whereas EPA and DHA are prudent in the production of healthy brain tissue, ALA is a powerful antioxidant that protects the brain. The harmful things that we eat and take in cause damage to healthy brain cells over time. This is known as neurodegeneration. While people can be genetically predisposed to neurodegenerative diseases, the onset and severity change with how much damage the brain experiences over a lifetime. ALA fights free radicals that cause damage to the brain (and other areas of the body). This prevents damage before it happens and helps maintain long-term brain health.

Fish Oil and Brain Health
Fish oil is among the many supplements that can improve brain function. In addition to its ability to work as fat in the body, it helps fight depression and mood problems that can make it hard to focus. Additionally, fish oil has been proven to improve memory in people who have difficulty remembering things.

Though there has been some debate about how much fish oil should be taken each day, the US Food & Drug Administration has recommended daily intake of 3,000 milligrams per day, while the European Food Safety Authority recommends a daily intake at or below 5,000 mg per day. You can supplement this amount by starting your day with a 1-2,000 mg capsule of fish oil and adding other sources of healthy fats to your diet.

One thing to note is that fish oil does not necessarily improve brain function if you are already healthy. However, most people have experienced cognitive degeneration through their life and may suffer from the presence of free radicals that cause damage in the brain. Even the foods you eat and the air you breathe may have chemicals that damage brain cells and functioning. The presence of disease and failing to get enough sleep can also cause a reduction in the number of healthy brain cells.

Something to note is that not all fish oil supplements are created equally. Supplements are not monitored by the FDA, as they are considered dietary rather than medicinal. As long as they are not harmful, there is no limit to the claims that can be made. As you consider supplements, choose a supplement that has been tested for mercury, toxins, and metals like arsenic and cadmium that may have contaminated a fish' living environment. Heavy metals are especially dangerous in humans, as they can cause loss or coordination, deafness, blindness, memory loss, irreversible damage to the kidney and liver, and even death. Polychlorinated biphenyls (PCBs), dioxins, and polybrominated biphenyls (PBBs) can also accumulate in fish. The ideal fish oil will come from fish species that have shorter lifespans, such as sardines, anchovies, and mackerel. These species also are not bottom feeders, so they do not consume as many contaminants. Then, the oil should still be purified before being bottled and sold to consumers.

Eating fish regularly is another way to get DHA and EPA. This is the most effective way, as the only plant sources are microalgae and seaweed and the fatty acids exist in very low concentrations. It would be hard to find a supplement that had high enough levels to boost brain health. ALA can also be eaten, rather than taken in supplement form. It is found in chia seeds, flax seeds, and walnuts in high levels. You can easily sprinkle these on top of a salad, put them in a smoothie, eat them on yogurt, or have a handful for a snack.

The Incredible Power of Antioxidants

Antioxidants are critical to brain health because they eliminate free radicals, which are a by-product of the body using oxygen. Free radicals typically attack and damage healthy cells—they can even cause autoimmune disorders or cancer. In the brain, free radicals can bounce around and damage healthy brain tissue, resulting in brain cell death and in some cases, neurodegeneration.

Free radicals develop in the body from exposure to your surroundings. They may develop from smoking cigarettes, using chemical cleaning products, and exposure to other toxins in the environment. Free radicals even result when your body breaks down certain foods within the body. While there are steps you can take to reduce your exposure to chemical-containing substances that result in free radicals, it is inevitable that you will come into contact with them in your environment. When these free radicals accumulate in the body, they begin to attack healthy cells. This can result in tumor growth, cancer, and even autoimmune disorders.

Antioxidants are known for their incredible ability to protect the cells of the body from damage caused by free radicals. Among these antioxidants are vitamins E and C, as well as carotenoids, flavonoids, tannins, lignans, and phenols. Generally, plant-based foods are among the best places to get antioxidants. This includes fruits and vegetables, seeds, nuts, spices and herbs, whole-grain products, and cocoa. Typically, you can expect the types of foods high in antioxidants to be high in fiber, low in cholesterol, and low in saturated fat. As they are available in a wide range of foods, there is a lot of potential to enjoy a variety of antioxidants.

You Don't Have to Avoid Sweets Completely- Eat Dark Chocolate in Moderation for a Brain Boost
Have you ever wondered why you feel so much better after letting a delicious bar of chocolate dissolve in your mouth? Chocolate is made from the cocoa bean, which contains tryptophan. Tryptophan is important for the production of serotonin. (You'll learn more about why this is important later). Dark chocolate is also full of antioxidants and flavonoids, both of which are important for fighting off free radicals that can damage healthy brain tissue and gray matter.

Another benefit of flavonoids is their ability to boost memory and improve cognitive functioning, as proven in a 2009 study by Oxford University. Something to keep in mind is that you need to choose dark chocolate with 70% cocoa for it to provide all the benefits. This might taste bitter if you are accustomed to sweeter kinds of chocolate, but you'll learn to appreciate it with time. In addition to all the benefits for the brain, studies have shown that dark chocolate benefits cardiovascular function, reducing the risk of stroke and heart disease and lowering blood pressure. You should also only eat dark chocolate in moderation, as it still contains a high amount of sugar and fat.

Other Antioxidant-Rich Foods

Among the many foods that you can eat to improve the level of antioxidants in your body are:

- Berries- Berries are one of the best sources of antioxidants, particularly blueberries, cranberries, blueberries, raspberries, and strawberries. While other fruits may have some antioxidants, berries contain the highest amount.
- Other Fruits- While not all other fruits will have the same antioxidant content as berries, there are plenty of options for getting a wide variety of antioxidants. This includes stone fruits like cherries, prunes, plums, nectarines, peaches, and apricots, most citrus fruits, grapes, apples with the peel on, olives, pomegranates, and tropical fruits like guava, banana, mango, and dates.
- Vegetables- There are several vegetable choices that can deliver a large number of antioxidants. The highest amounts come from bell peppers, artichokes, and kale, which was mentioned earlier. Other antioxidant-rich veggies include red cabbage, beets, asparagus, and broccoli.
- Tomatoes- Tomatoes are another produce item that deserves a special mention. Tomatoes contain the antioxidant lycopene, which prevents free radical damage. One study found lycopene an effective antioxidant in preventing Alzheimer's. If you are trying to get your full intake of lycopene, keep in mind that it is most beneficial when it is released from the fiber of fresh tomatoes. If you buy a tomato paste, the ingredients will be more bioavailable.

- Sweet Potatoes- Sweet potatoes are full of antioxidants that help keep your brain protected from free radicals. In addition to antioxidants, they are full of key vitamins, fiber, and healthy carbohydrates. These work together and slowly release the sugars into your bloodstream, meaning your brain stays energized longer. The sweet potato also contains Vitamin C and beta-carotene, which is the precursor to Vitamin A. Darker sweet potatoes have a higher level of antioxidants, but all sweet potatoes contain 16 anthocyanins, a beneficial brain antioxidant.
- Nuts- Nuts have been mentioned for their incredible healthy fat content. Those that have the most antioxidants as well are pecans, almonds, hazelnuts, pistachios, and walnuts. Ground flaxseed, sesame seeds, and sunflower seeds are also full of antioxidants.
- Legumes- Legumes include beans, lentils, and edamame. Kidney beans are among those with the highest level of antioxidants. You can eat edamame salted, add beans to rice, or make a lentil soup.
- Beverages- There are several drinks that you can have with antioxidant benefits, including the coffee or tea that you start your morning with. Red wine, pomegranate juice, and berry juices are also good choices. It is important to keep in mind that there are different types of antioxidants in everything—variety is the best way to be sure you are getting all of them.
- Green Tea- Green tea has incredible antioxidant benefits. It has one of the highest known amounts of the flavonoid catechins—it is the antioxidant equivalent of eating 8 apples! The antioxidants in

green tea are also easily absorbed by the body, which allows them to be used properly.

As you make the switch to a better diet, you'll find that getting the nutrients you need to preserve and maintain brain health becomes easier. Nutrition is also something that becomes easier with time. Your motivation will be supercharged as you experience higher energy levels, better digestive health, an increased ability to focus, and a general feeling of wellness. As your mind becomes less addicted to the harmful foods you ate before, you'll be less likely to crave them and eating healthy becomes effortless.

Chapter 6: Eat Fat, Lose Weight

As mentioned earlier, the Ketogenic diet is among those that has gained popularity for its low-carb, high-fat regiment that helps you lose weight. Typically, the body burns available carbohydrates as energy. When you are trying to lose weight, however, this does not tap into the fat stores of the body to produce the results you are looking for. This chapter will discuss the science of losing weight with fat, as well as provide some examples of good fats that you can include in your diet.

The Science behind a Low-Carb, High-Fat Diet

At one time, many people believed that a low-fat diet was the key to making your body get rid of accumulated. However, despite the rise of low-fat diets, the obesity rate has continued to rise. This is because we are still working to understand exactly how the body works. Recently, the idea of eating fats to become thin has become popular because of its effects on key hormones in the body.

When you eat carbohydrate-rich foods or those that are high in refined grains or sugar, your bloodstream fills with insulin. The problem with insulin is that its release also sends the message to fat cells that they must extract the fat cells from the blood and store them for later. By contrast, when you keep your insulin levels low, that signal to store fat is not being sent.

Insulin also impacts the influence of leptin, which is known as the hunger hormone. When leptin increases in the body, it causes your body to feel full and satisfied. When you eat high levels of carbohydrates, the insulin that your body releases dominates the signal from the leptin. This can cause you to crave more food and carbohydrates.

As you continue to eat fat, it can also improve your weight loss efforts because it makes your body more sensitive to insulin. This means that when you do eat carbohydrates, your bloodstream is not flooded with insulin. Instead, your body releases less insulin to deal with the same amount of carbohydrates, which stops extreme spikes in blood sugar.

One team of researchers at Harvard followed the weight loss efforts of 101 men and women for 18 months. Of the groups, half were on a low-fat diet and the other half were on a diet that had approximately 20% of daily caloric consumption from monounsaturated fatty acids, which are those beneficial to brain health. Some of the sources of fats used during the study include safflower oil, nuts, olives, and avocados. Of the participants in the study, those who ate the higher fat diet lost an average of 11 pounds and kept them off, while the low-fat group lost only an average of 6 pounds. This would make it ideal for people trying to lose weight while boosting brain health to reduce the consumption of sugars and carbohydrates. Additionally, about half of daily calories should come from healthy fats and lean proteins.

How Eating Healthy Fat Helps You Lose Weight
The body needs a set number of calories to have the energy it needs. While something like protein is vital to bodily function, you can vary the amount of fat or carbohydrates that you eat and still get the fuel you need.

The three major macronutrients that the body needs to function are fat, carbohydrates, and protein. When you eat more fat, you eat fewer carbohydrates to compensate. Likewise, eating more carbohydrates means eating less fat.

When you adjust the number of fats vs. carbohydrates you are eating, it changes the amount of insulin released by your body. You can think of insulin as the gatekeeper of the body's nutrients. It hoards nutrients in the fat stores of your body. When you reduce carbohydrates, your body releases less insulin. This allows it to access fat stores and transport them to the muscles and tissue through the body, effectively fueling your body with fat.

The problem that happens with many low-fat diets that were once popular was the negative impact on adipokines, especially the hormone adiponectin that is released from fat cells. When released, adiponectin works to burn fat, increasing metabolism and curbing appetite. When you do not eat enough fats, you do not have enough adiponectin to maintain a healthy metabolism.

In addition to helping your body burn fat better, eating fats satiates your appetite. Once your body processes it and the fat enters the small intestine, it signals to the body with the release of the hormones PYY (peptide YY) and CCK (cholecystokinin). These are critical in sending signals that you are satiated, which makes it less likely that you are going to eat a second helping or eat extra snacks through the day.

Choosing Good Fats

Among the good fats that you include in your diet, try including these food choices:

- Avocado- Avocado is rich in omega-3 fatty acids. They are also a good source of potassium and Vitamin E. You can eat it with some salt, put it on a sandwich, or make guacamole by mashing it and adding lime juice and diced tomato.
- Fish- Fish oil is often taken as a supplement to promote brain health. Regularly consuming fish can also ensure you are getting enough good fats in your diet. Fresh salmon, trout, herring, and tuna are ideal, but tinned salmon and mackerel also have a sufficient amount of healthy fats. You should try to eat three portions of oily fish per week to get enough good oils.
- Nuts and seeds- Most nuts and seeds contain some type of oil, each of them rich in omega-3s and omega-6s. If you don't want to eat a handful of nuts, there are plenty of other options. Add nuts to your cereal, sprinkle them on yogurt, or use them to give your salad an extra crunch. Nuts and seeds are also good sources of fiber and protein.
- Oils- Walnut oil and canola oil have a high level of omega-3s, as well as omega-6's. This allows them to provide the balance that is important to maintain both heart and brain health.
- Nut Butters- Nut butters are full of healthy fats and protein, as well as key vitamins and minerals. They can be spread on whole grain toast, eaten with celery or apples, or added to a smoothie for a nutty kick.

As with many of the other food groups, you should work to combine a wide variety of fats in your diet. Variety will ensure you have a healthy balance of fats, encouraging both brain and heart health. It is also important to remember that you must decrease carbohydrates while you increase fats. Otherwise, you will end up gaining weight as your body tries to run off two separate fuel sources.

Diet to Lose Weight with Fat

If you look up 'low-fat' diet online, you are going to be bombarded with the dozens of diets that exist. Unless you have a degree in food science or nutrition, it can be difficult to consider which of these diets will be most beneficial for your body. This is especially true because nearly all of them have some doctor or famous personality vouching for their effectiveness.

The Ketogenic diet mentioned in the last chapter is one of the diets that will boost brain health while helping you lose weight. The key to finding success with this diet is balancing the number of fats and carbs that you eat for your body. If you want to lose weight with a high-fat diet, there is another alternative. There are many basic diets that involve eating fat. To stop your body from going into shock, as it might when you suddenly switch to a Ketogenic diet, you should transition slowly.

Deciding Your Caloric Needs
Before you get started, you'll need to figure out how many calories you should be consuming each day. The average woman needs 2000 calories per day to maintain their weight, while the average man needs 2500 calories per day for weight maintenance. For weight loss, a woman needs 1500 calories and a man needs 2000 calories each day to lose one pound each week. Even though these are averages, the specific caloric amount you need each day is affected by several factors. In addition to gender, a person's current weight, metabolic health, age, height,

and activity levels come into play. There are many calculators available online that can help you decide how many calories you need based on these factors.

The Easy-Transition Diet
Once you know how many calories you need, you'll calculate how much of each type of macronutrient you should be getting from your food. For the first two weeks, your diet should be 50% fat, 25% protein, and 25% carbohydrates. This means that a man trying to eat a 2000-calorie per day diet to lose weight would consume 1000 calories from fat, 500 calories from protein, and 500 calories from carbohydrates. Even though you should consume carbohydrates during this phase, you should avoid carbohydrates from added sugars, grain products, and starchy potatoes. Instead, get carbohydrates from legumes, beans, and fruits. Cutting out grain and sugars altogether will help curb your cravings by going cold turkey.

The length of the second phase is going to depend on the amount of weight you are trying to lose. It is generally recommended that you complete this from several weeks up to six months, then give yourself a break before dieting again if you have not yet reached your weight loss goal. During this phase, 40% of your calories will come from fat, 35% will come from carbohydrates, and 25% will come from protein. You do not have to avoid grains completely during this phase. However, you should stick to those that slow-digesting carbohydrates that will not send your insulin skyrocketing. This includes oats, quinoa, and brown rice.

You should enter the final phase when you are ready to maintain your weight. Not only is this diet easy to follow, but it is also perfect for providing your brain with the fats it needs to thrive. This ratio is similar to the Mediterranean diet. The typical daily diet should come from 20% protein, 40% carbohydrates, and 40% fat. If you go six months on phase two of the diet without losing all the weight you want, you should transition to phase three for one month while you let your body reset. Then, return to phase two for as long as you need to meet your weight loss goal.

Optional: The Cleansing Phase
Something that many people do before beginning a diet is a cleansing phase. While it is optional, you are encouraged to do it. This is especially true if you eat a diet that is high in sugar, alcohol, carbohydrates, processed ingredients, or other unhealthy foods. Doing a cleanse is also incredibly beneficial for the digestive tract. It clears the digestive environment of harmful elements and paves the way for healthy, beneficial bacteria to thrive. This will increase nutrient absorption and help you get the most benefits from the foods you are eating and the supplements you are taking.

The cleansing phase involves two parts. The first major part involves cleansing your household and setting yourself up for success. There is no reason to challenge yourself more than necessary by keeping unhealthy foods in your house. If unhealthy foods are not always immediately accessible, it gives you time to think about the decision to eat foods and if it is really worth it. You should remove products with refined flour, those that are high in sugar or sodium, and foods that are generally unhealthy to eat. Look over the list of some of the worst foods for you—then remove those things from your refrigerator and pantry.

You should avoid doing diet cleanses sold on the shelves or doing anything too extreme to cleanse. One thing that can help naturally clean out your digestive tract is drinking plenty of water and fiber-rich juices. You should also eat plenty of vegetables. During the cleansing phase, you should limit your intake of carbohydrates from grain sources and avoid processed foods. Adding a little lemon juice to water or taking a tablespoon of apple cider vinegar are also known to help remove waste from the body.

Add Fats, but Beware of Calories
If you are adding fat to your diet in an effort to lose weight, you cannot do so with reckless abandon. After all, fast foods are full of fats—but they are also full of carbohydrates, processed ingredients, and other unhealthy foods for your body. Even too many healthy fats can be a bad thing. They can drastically increase your number of calories and while you can be sure your brain is getting enough fat to encourage its health, it can also accumulate in fat deposits around your body.

Chapter 7: Brain Boosting Super-Herbs and Nootropics

Nootropics were discovered by Dr. Giurgea when he was studying a synthetic drug called Piracetam, which combatted mental problems like schizophrenia and dementia. Interestingly, it was able to bring balance and stability to the mind, whether it was overactive like in the case of schizophrenia or underactive like in the case of dementia. This study helped lead to an understanding of nootropics, which are natural enhancers for various abilities.

The History of Nootropics

The idea of having a miracle drug to make someone 'smarter' is not a new concept. People naturally want to be physically and mentally better. It is something that drives athletes to compete to be the best and pushes chess players and puzzle solvers to enter in a competition. Even though the idea of being the best is not new, the concept of nootropics has existed for less than a century.

As a drug, the first nootropic was developed in the 1960s for motion sickness. The first study on this drug (called piracetam) as a nootropic was done in 1971. The term 'nootropic' was coined by Dr. Corneliu Giurgea of Romania, derived from the Greek words 'nous' (mind) and 'trepein' (to bend). The way that they 'bent' the mind described their ability to improve the way that the mind functioned.

Even though Dr. Giurgea is credited with coining the term 'nootropics', these beneficial herbs have been around since the beginning of medicine. They were used by Native Americans and practitioners of Ayurveda and Traditional Chinese Medicine to promote healing and balance, especially following a brain injury. Though the recent history and studying nootropics using Western science is new, comparatively, the ancient history of these super herbs speaks volumes to their safety and effectiveness.

Natural Nootropics: What Are They

Natural nootropics are natural supplements that have different effects on the mind. They increase your overall cognitive potential, bringing balance in your focus and attention. They also can improve motivation, learning ability, creativity, and memory. Physically, nootropics improve circulation in the brain, reduce neuroinflammation, and have neuroprotective benefits. They also work by creating stronger connections between the neurons of the brain, helping you reach a greater level of comprehension and understanding of the world. Here are some of the major benefits of nootropics:

- Increased Motivation- By enhancing your desire to do things, you can increase your mental strength and endurance. As the connections between neurons in your brain grow stronger, it increases your physical and mental potential.

- Activation of Natural Energy- Nootropics nourish the body and activate your natural energy stores. You'll find that your body and mind are ready for anything that you need to do—whether you work eight hours or twelve.

- Increased Focus- Some people use prescription drugs to increase their focus, particularly those who struggle with ADHD. The problem is that many of these drugs cause side effects like difficulty sleeping, trouble eating, and sweaty palms. Nootropics enhance focus by increasing your mind's capacity for attention.

- Improved Short-Term Memory- The amino acids and vitamins found in nootropics stimulate the production of chemicals that promote short-term retention and memory gain.

- Improved Long-Term Memory- The stimulation caused by nootropics encourage the neurotransmitters of the brain to work in sync. Your brain becomes capable of gathering more data, which forms stronger memories.

- Decreased Brain Fog- Have you ever found yourself staring at a task, not realizing that you are looking at it without working? This is called brain fog. It is a time where you cannot keep your mind focused, even when you are not distracted by something else. Nootropics give you the mental energy you need to stay focused all day long.

- Creative Thinking- Nootropics increase your creativity by enhancing your brain power. You will find yourself considering new possibilities and thinking more deeply about things. This fresh perspective allows you to become more innovative, helping propel you to success.

How Nootropics Work

Some nootropics are natural, while others are lab-created. While the two work in the same way, the nootropics discussed in this chapter will be derived from natural ingredients. Nootropics work by improving the overall health of the brain. They are involved in many critical processes, including oxidation, brain inflammation, and blood circulation.

Think of it this way. In the body, there are many tiny vessels that run from your heart to your brain. These vessels are responsible for carrying blood full of oxygen and vital nutrients to your brain. Additionally, these same vessels transport toxins, waste, hormones, and neurotransmitters from the brain. This encourages brain health and allows the brain to send messages to all other areas of the body.

When the vessels become inflamed, they become constricted. This limits the amount of blood that can flow from the brain to the rest of the body and from the rest of the body to the brain. In some people, this inflammation results in a brain fog. In others, this flow occurs over time and it causes a slow death of brain cells. This can cause neurodegenerative conditions like dementia and Alzheimer's in the long-term.

Brain-Boosting Super-Herbs and Nootropics

1. L-Theanine- This nootropic is found in Matcha and green tea. It works to relax the brain, without making it tired or causing sedation. L-Theanine improves sleep quality, enhances mental activities, reduces anxiety, and increases your overall sense of well-being. It works by

boosting the levels of different neurotransmitters in the brain, including serotonin, GABA, glycine, and dopamine. It works well with stimulants like caffeine since it reduces anxiety.

2. Caffeine- Caffeine improves mental focus because of its anti-sleep abilities. As you wake up, your ability to focus increases and you can come out of a mental fog. The reason caffeine works is because of its ability to overcome the adenosine in the receptors. The adenosine slows down your brain, giving it time to store memories and replete its energy stores. This is the reason that many people experience a coffee crash sometime in the afternoon, once the caffeine has worn off.

3. Rhodiola- This is a well-known herb in Traditional Chinese Medicine. It increases cognitive and physical vitality. One of the ways Rhodiola works is by reducing mental fatigue, which promotes mental clarity through your day. It also boosts concentration and stimulates AMPK enzymes, which increases cognitive energy, boosts metabolic activity, and improves cell functioning. It also reduces stress and fatigue and balances mood and depression. Additionally, it works by increasing the levels of dopamine and serotonin in the brain. If your stomach feels upset after taking Rhodiola, try taking it with food. Some people do experience anxiety as well—Gotu Kola or Bacopa might be a better alternative if Rhodiola makes you anxious. It is also very stimulating, so avoid taking it right before bed.

4. Omega-3s- We have already mentioned the many benefits of Omega-3s. They are also incredible nootropics, improving cognition, encouraging cardiovascular health boosting mood, and reducing inflammation to protect the

brain. This comes from the key ingredients DHA (Docosahexaenoic Acid) and EPA (Eicosapentaenoic Acid). Some of the best Omega-3 supplements come from algae, krill, or fish oil. The results on EPA as a brain booster are mixed, however, it plays a critical role in preventing inflammation and aging effects that harm brain cells and volume. DHA has been proven effective at boosting the brain, likely because it makes up 90% of the omega-3 fat found in brain cells. It maintains the structure and functioning of the brain, as well as boosts thinking skills, reaction times, and memory recall.

5. Ginseng- Among ginseng's many abilities are increased exercise performance and testosterone levels boosted mood and increased cognitive abilities. Ginseng also helps fight against mental fatigue and increases happiness and perceived well-being. Additionally, ginseng boosts brain health (and other health) by improving blood flow and the movement of nutrients and oxygen through the body. Something to keep in mind is that there are more than one species of ginseng, with the most common being Panax Ginseng and American Ginseng. It is deeply rooted in Traditional Chinese and Ayurvedic medicine. Among the many mental benefits, ginseng stops inflammation that can harm the brain and has been proven in several studies to treat conditions of the mind including ADHD, Alzheimer's disease, and age-related neurodegeneration.

6. Citicoline- This is a precursor to the neurotransmitter acetylcholine and produces choline in the body, which is essential to processes like concentration, memory, and learning. Some of the best food sources for citicoline are beets, spinach, eggs, peanuts, and liver. Even though choline is essential for health, the USDA reports that an average of 60% of people is deficient. In addition to

working with acetylcholine, citicoline works with dopamine to protect the brain, preventing damage by oxidative stress and free radicals. It also encourages the regeneration and repair of membranes and connections between brain cells. In addition to getting choline from food sources, it is found in seaweed. Research from a team in Switzerland shows that taking a chlorella supplement derived from green algae provides long-term improvements in overall mental drive and memory recall while boosting attention span. It is also full of antioxidants that support healthy brain tissue and fight damaging free radicals.

7. Curcumin- Turmeric contains high levels of the active ingredient curcumin, which has several whole-body benefits. Its anti-inflammatory abilities allow it to fight against disease like cancer, metabolic syndrome, heart disease, Alzheimer's, and other degenerative conditions. It also repairs damage. It is important to note that the bioavailability of capsules and supplements is not very high, so it is best to consume curcumin with food instead.

8. Teacrine- Teacrine has a similar structure to caffeine, having the ability to boost energy, reduce tiredness, and fight off mental fatigue. It is commonly found in Kucha tea. Unlike coffee, it releases slower in the body and sustains its energy release, which helps prevent the coffee crash associated with caffeine. Another benefit of Teacrine over caffeine is that it does not store in the body and create a tolerance like caffeine. You will not have to increase the dosages over time, which means you will not face unwanted side effects like difficulty sleeping, anxiety, shakiness, and the jitters.

9. Pycnogenol- Also called pine bark extract, this nootropic improves blood sugar levels, increases blood flow, and reduces oxidative stress that causes damage to cells. Pycnogenol comes from the French maritime pine tree. Its benefits come mainly from its antioxidant properties, which stop damage to brain cells, delay the onset of cognitive decline, and have anti-aging benefits that encourage cognitive protection.

10. Brahmi- Brahmi (also called Bacopa Monierri) has a deep history in Ayurvedic medicine, being used for thousands of years to boost memory and learning, as well as treat anxiety. It encourages calmness like L-Theanine while enhancing memory abilities. Bacopa has also been proven to enhance visual processing, improve concentration, and improve memory. It also blocks stress signals in the brain, which stops the stress response from triggering and prevents anxiety altogether. The final way Brahmi enhances the brain is by increasing the enzyme TPH2. This helps create new connections between neurons in the brain and improves long-term memory by boosting the conversion of L-Tryptophan to serotonin.

11. Cordyceps Sinensis- Also referred to as Chinese Caterpillar Mushroom, this beneficial plant has been used as a tonic in Indian, Chinese, and Tibetan cultures. It boosts focus and increases mental energy. This herb first came to light in Western medicine in 1993, when two Chinese women beat the world records in the Stuttgart World Championships for running. Their supplement and training regimen were credited for the women's intense focus and ability to excel at track and field.

12. CoQ10- Coenzyme Quinone is a powerful antioxidant that fights against the natural aging processes of the body

and the cells. It can protect the brain from the effects of aging and plays a critical role in creating energy in the mitochondria. It is natural for the body to slow down its production of CoQ10 with time, which is one of the reasons the brain and cells are less protected from the effects of aging. While there are some food sources of CoQ10, most contain trace amounts of the nutrient that make it impossible to consume enough food to experience the benefits. For example, you would need to eat several buckets of broccoli or 133 cups of cabbage to get the daily recommended amount. This is a case where taking a supplement is a more practical option.

13. Niacin- The B-vitamins are known for their role in energy and how they are involved in various functions through the body. However, Niacin (vitamin B3) stands out for its effectiveness as a nootropic. Not only does niacin play a critical role in converting food to energy, but it also works as a catalyst when neurotransmitters are being created in the brain. By making this process more efficient, it streamlines the use of energy. Vitamin B3 also transforms fats, proteins, and carbohydrates into energy and synthesizes glycogen in the muscles and liver for energy use. This encourages the process of ketosis and prevents the body from eating away at the tissues when it becomes tired or runs low on energy supplies.

14. Gotu Kola- Gotu Kola has documented use in India for the last 2,500 years. It is considered a memory tonic, with Sanskrit texts reading that drinking the juice of Gotu Kola boosts memory and cognitive abilities after just one week. In the long-term, it is believed to enhance an individual's photographic memory and promote a longer lifespan. One way that it does this is because of its effects on the neurotransmitter gamma-aminobutyric acid (GABA).

GABA is associated with relaxation, which is beneficial for promoting relaxation. Gotu Kola boosts mental focus because of its properties as an adaptogen, which relaxes without causing sleepiness. It also works to reduce anxiety and has antioxidant benefits that fight free radicals that damage healthy brain tissue.

14. Lion's Mane- Lion's Mane is a plant used in Traditional Chinese Medicine, being a mushroom that works by promoting the growth of nerves in the brain. By inducing nerve growth factor, Lion's Mane improves cognition by healing nerve damage. It may even reduce symptoms of a brain injury or harm caused by deterioration from conditions like dementia, Alzheimer's disease, muscular dystrophy, and Parkinson's disease. Lion's Mane also has antioxidants that reduce oxidative stress. Additionally, it improves focus and helps balance mood, particularly in people who struggle with depression.

15. Bacopa- This is an herb known for its powerful effects because of Ayurvedic medicine. Like Gotu Kola, this is calming but will not make you drowsy. Its primary use is to boost focus and increase memory. Studies have shown that it can improve memory in people of any age. Additionally, some studies point to its effectiveness in decreasing the progression of neurodegenerative disease and helps people who are recovering from brain trauma. Though it is an adaptogen that promotes a feeling of calmness, Bacopa heals best when used for several months. It provides support for the immune system, reduces the effects of stress through the body, and is an antioxidant that protects the brain while promoting healthy neural blood flow and the production of neurotransmitters. This is an especially bitter herb that

can cause stomach upset, so try taking it with food if you need to.

Should You Use Nootropics?

When you decide to take nootropics, there is little to lose. These herbs are non-toxic in the human body. They work in a natural way to promote healthy brain function, improve memory, reduces stress, and benefit the way that you think. This improved ability of the brain's functioning gives you the opportunity to excel in life.

As you choose a nootropic supplement, keep in mind that they are not always created equal. It is important to choose a supplement that has been tested for contaminants to ensure you are not taking anything that will harm your health. In addition to looking for something that has been third-party tested, consider how the herb is processed. Some manufacturers heat the nootropics and herbs to process them. Heating at high temperatures can kill the beneficial components. Finding supplements that have been pressed or undergone carbon dioxide pressing is a better option.

Conclusion

When was the last time you thought about what your food choices are doing for you? When something as simple as nutrition has the power to increase the quality of your life, the only logical thing to do is improve your diet. Hopefully, this book has taught you all that you need to know to eat in a way that encourages brain health. By cutting out harmful substances and eating a diet high in healthy fats, antioxidant-rich fruits and vegetables, and nootropics, you can preserve the health of your brain through your life.

For many people, the thing holding them back from success is their mind. By encouraging your health on a cellular level, you can fight off chronic and degenerative diseases. You can also improve your focus and memory, increase your energy levels, encourage the growth of new connections in your brain, and so much more. Every food that you eat and supplement that you take has the potential to harm or help your brain health. By choosing healthy fats avoiding the foods that harm your brain, and choosing foods that benefit the mitochondria, you can improve your mental and physical health.

Now that you have this information available, you have everything you need to start eating the right fuels for your brain. The only logical 'next step' is to get started!

Resources

https://www.health.harvard.edu/blog/nutritional-psychiatry-your-brain-on-food-201511168626

https://www.healthline.com/health/mental-health/serotonin#functions

https://www.psychologytoday.com/us/articles/200310/what-is-good-brain-food

https://www.npr.org/2011/03/24/132745785/how-western-diets-are-making-the-world-sick

https://www.hopkinsmedicine.org/health/healthy_aging/healthy_body/the-brain-gut-connection

https://www.healthline.com/nutrition/probiotics-and-weight-loss#section

https://healthfully.com/440659-is-egg-a-brain-food.html

https://www.topuniversities.com/blog/foods-fuel-brain

https://www.wgu.edu/blog/brain-fuel-5-food-groups-successful-students1712.html#openSubscriberModal

https://healthfully.com/358464-antioxidants-in-dark-chocolate.html

https://www.psychologytoday.com/us/articles/200310/what-is-good-brain-food

https://www.mayoclinic.org/healthy-lifestyle/nutrition-and-healthy-eating/multimedia/antioxidants/sls-20076428

https://neurotrition.ca/blog/brain-food-essentials-sweet-potato

https://www.amazing-green-tea.com/green-tea-antioxidants.html

https://www.livestrong.com/article/22253-foods-high-b-vitamins/

https://www.livescience.com/50818-kale-nutrition.html

http://www.learninginfo.org/food-for-the-brain.htm

https://www.rd.com/health/diet-weight-loss/eat-healthy-fats-to-lose-weight/

https://www.myfooddata.com/articles/high-tryptophan-foods.php

https://www.healthline.com/nutrition/11-super-healthy-probiotic-foods#section12

https://www.psychologytoday.com/intl/blog/you-illuminated/201010/why-your-brain-needs-water

https://www.eatthis.com/drink-water-lose-weight/

https://www.forbes.com/sites/alicegwalton/2016/12/09/7-ways-sleep-affects-the-brain-and-what-happens-if-it-doesnt-get-enough/

https://www.psychologytoday.com/us/blog/the-athletes-way/201404/physical-activity-improves-cognitive-function

https://www.shape.com/lifestyle/mind-and-body/why-sleep-no-1-most-important-thing-better-body

https://www.mayoclinic.org/healthy-lifestyle/fitness/in-depth/exercise/art-20048389

https://www.ncbi.nlm.nih.gov/pubmed/27836629

https://mitochondrialdiseasenews.com/2015/11/23/mitochondria-linked-psychological-stress-response-study/

https://www.umdf.org/what-is-mitochondrial-disease/

https://www.healthline.com/nutrition/worst-foods-for-your-brain#section1

https://www.thebestbrainpossible.com/how-to-optimize-your-mitochondria-for-a-healthier-brain/

https://www.bewell.com/blog/care-keeping-mitochondria/

http://eatdrinkpaleo.com.au/the-best-foods-for-mitochondrial-health/

https://www.healthline.com/nutrition/low-carb-ketogenic-diet-brain

https://www.masteringdiabetes.org/what-are-ketones/

https://www.health.harvard.edu/mind-and-mood/protect-your-brain-with-good-fat

https://www.livescience.com/20429-good-fats-good-brain.html

https://www.webmd.com/diet/features/eat-smart-healthier-brain#1

https://www.healthline.com/nutrition/omega-3-fish-oil-for-brain-health#section4

https://www.dmarge.com/2018/03/need-eat-fat-order-lose-weight.html

https://www.thedailybeast.com/eat-fat-lose-weight-the-anti-hunger-diet

https://articles.mercola.com/sites/articles/archive/2017/04/24/burning-fat-for-fuel.aspx

https://www.eatthebutter.org/fat-makes-you-thin/

https://www.naturalstacks.com/blogs/news/the-ultimate-resource-for-nootropics

https://blog.gethapi.me/10-brain-boosting-superherbs-and-natural-nootropics-to-kickstart-your-day-e389be453b2d
https://www.verywellmind.com/what-is-the-fight-or-flight-response-2795194
https://www.tuw.edu/health/how-stress-affects-the-brain/
https://www.sciencedaily.com/releases/2012/08/120812151659.htm
https://www.scientificamerican.com/article/stress-kills-brain-cells/
https://www.sciencedaily.com/releases/2014/09/140918091418.htm
http://www.medicinalgenomics.com/wp-content/uploads/2011/12/Mitochondria_Ox-Stress_Neurology.pdf
https://www.ncbi.nlm.nih.gov/pmc/articles/PMC4566449/
https://www.businessinsider.com/what-happens-when-you-dont-get-enough-sleep-2017-12
https://howtobrain.com/using-omega-3s-for-brain-healing/
https://www.lifesdha.com/en_US/news/why-the-brain-needs-omega-3-fatty-acids.html
https://www.forbes.com/sites/michaelpellmanrowland/2017/06/26/cheese-addiction/#3d4e39c23583
https://www.healthline.com/nutrition/how-to-overcome-food-addiction#first-steps
https://www.ncbi.nlm.nih.gov/pubmed/18072818
https://drhoffman.com/article/what-are-epadha-13/
http://glutathionepro.com/enhancing-brain-health-acetyl-l-carnitine-alpha-lipoic-acid/
https://www.brainmdhealth.com/blog/choose-good-fish-oil/

https://www.ruled.me/guide-keto-diet/
https://dailyburn.com/life/health/always-hungry-david-ludwig-diet/
https://www.bodybuilding.com/content/how-eating-more-fat-helps-you-lose-more-weight.html
https://www.healthline.com/nutrition/how-many-calories-per-day
https://www.livestrong.com/article/107334-cleanse-body-before-dieting/
https://www.endocrineweb.com/conditions/hyperglycemia/hyperglycemia-when-your-blood-glucose-level-goes-too-high
https://www.ruled.me/ketogenic-diet-food-list/
https://www.ruled.me/ketogenic-diet-epilepsy/
https://www.purenootropics.net/general-nootropics/history-of-nootropics/
http://www.brain-smart.net/top-4-natural-nootropics-to-improve-your-brain-health/#axzz5iaIyhoVW
https://lostempireherbs.com/nootropic-herbs-for-brain-health/
https://www.healthline.com/nutrition/best-nootropic-brain-supplements
https://ubiquinol.org/blog/six-incredible-ways-get-ubiquinol-coq10-food
https://draxe.com/ginseng-benefits/

www.ingramcontent.com/pod-product-compliance
Lightning Source LLC
Chambersburg PA
CBHW030727180526
45157CB00008BA/3081